GLUTEN FREE
FOOD LIST

The World's Most Comprehensive Ingredient List for
the Gluten-Free Diet - Take It Wherever You Go!

MORGAN F. WHITTAKER

LEGAL & DISCLAIMER

Contents

LEGAL & DISCLAIMER 1

CONTENTS 3

INTRODUCTION.. 19

HOW TO USE THIS FOOD LIST 23

LEGAL DEFINITIONS OF 'GLUTEN-FREE'... 25

SOURCES 27

DISCLAIMER 29

THE FOOD LIST 31

Acerola 31

Agave syrup... 31

Alcohol 31

Algae and algae derivatives.. 31

Almond 31

Amaranth... 32

Anchovies 32

Anise, aniseed 32

Apple 32

Apple cider vinegar... 32

Apricot... 33

Artichoke 33
Artificial sweeteners 33
Asimina triloba 33
Asparagus 33
Aubergine 33
Avocado 33
Bamboo shoots 33
Banana 34
Barbary fig 34
Barley 34
Barley malt, malt 34
Basil 34
Bay laurel, laurel 34
Beans (pulses) 34
Beef (depending on age of beef, organic, freshly
cooked) 35
Beer 35
Beetroot 35
Bell pepper (hot) 35
Bell pepper (sweet) 35
Bison (organic, freshly cooked) 35
Bivalves (mussels, oyster, clams, scallops) 35
Black caraway 36
Black caraway oil 36
Blackberry 36
Blackcurrants 36
Blue cheeses, mold cheeses 36
Blue fenugreek 36

Blueberries 36
Bok choi 36
Borlotti beans 36
Bouillon (yeast extract / meat extract / glutamate) 36
Boysenberry... 37
Brandy 37
Brazil nut 37
Bread 37
Broad bean... 37
Broad-leaved garlic 37
Broccoli 37
Brown algae, algae 37
Brussels sprouts 38
Buckrams.. 38
Buckwheat.. 38
Butter 38
Butterkaese 38
Buttermilk... 38
Cabbage, green or white 38
Cactus pear 39
Caraway 39
Cardamom 39
Carrot... 39
Cashew nut... 39
Cassava 39
Cassava flour.. 39
Cauliflower 39
Celery 40

Celery cabbage 40
Cep 40
Chamomile tea... 40
Champagne 40
Chard stalks... 40
Chayote.. 40
Cheddar cheese 40
Cheese made from unpasteurised "raw" milk 41
Cheese: soft cheeses.. 41
Cheese: hard cheese, all well matured cheeses.................... 41
Cherry 41
Chestnut, sweet chestnut... 41
Chia 41
Chicken 41
Chickpeas 42
Chicory... 42
Chili pepper, red, fresh 42
Chives.. 42
Chocolate... 42
Cilantro 43
Cinnamon 43
Citrus fruits.. 43
Clover 43
Cloves.. 43
Cocoa butter 43
Cocoa drinks.. 43
Cocoa, cocoa powder (chocolate, etc.)...................... 44
Coconut fat, coconut oil... 44

Coconut, coconut shavings, coconut milk 44
Coffee 44
Cola-drinks 44
Common sea-buckthorn 45
Coriander 45
Corn 45
Corn salad, lamb's lettuce 45
Cornflakes (if no additives) 45
Courgette 46
Cowberry 46
Crab 46
Cranberry 46
Cranberry nectar 46
Crawfish 46
Cream cheeses (means: very young cheeses), plain,
without additives 46
Cream, sweet, without additives 47
Cress: garden cress 47
Cucumber 47
Cumin 47
Curd cheese 47
Curry 47
Dates (dried, desiccated) 47
Dextrose 48
Dill 48
Distilled white vinegar 48
Dog rose 48
Dragon fruit, pitaya 48

Dried meat (any kind) 48

Dry-cured ham 48

Duck 49

Earth almond 49

Egg white 49

Egg yolk 49

Eggplant 49

Eggs, chicken egg, whole egg 49

Elderflower cordial 49

Elderflower cordial 50

Endive 50

Energy drinks 50

Entrails 50

Espresso 50

Ethanol 50

Ewe's milk, sheep's milk 51

Extract of malt 51

Farmer's cheese (a type of fresh cheese) 51

Fennel 51

Fennel flower (Nigella sativa) 51

Fennel flower oil (Nigella sativa) 51

Fenugreek 51

Feta cheese 51

Figs (fresh or dried) 52

Fish (freshly caught within an hour or frozen within
an hour) 52

Fish (in the shop in the cooling rack or on ice) 52

Flaxseed (linseed) 52

Fontina cheese.. 52
Fries, chips... 52
Fructose (fruit sugar)... 53
Game.. 53
Garden cress 53
Garlic (usually well tolerated).. 53
Geheimratskaese, Geheimrats cheese 53
German turnip 53
Ginger 53
Glucose 54
Goat's milk, goat milk.. 54
Goji berry, Chinese wolfberry, Chinese boxthorn,
Himalayan goji, Tibetan goji 54
Goose (organic, freshly cooked) 54
Gooseberry, gooseberries... 54
Gouda cheese (young) 54
Gouda cheese, old.. 54
Gourds 54
Grapefruit.. 55
Grapes.. 55
Gravy 55
Green algae, algae.. 55
Green beans 55
Green peas 55
Green split peas.. 55
Green tea.. 56
Guava 56
Ham (dried, cured) 56

4

Hazelnut... 56
Hemp seeds (Cannabis sativa)..................................... 56
Herbal teas with medicinal herbs................................ 56
Honey... 56
Horseradish.. 57
Hot chocolate.. 57
Indian fig opuntia, Barbary fig, cactus pear, spineless
cactus, prickly pear, tuna... 57
Innards... 57
Inverted sugar syrup... 57
Ispaghula, psyllium seed husks 57
Jeera (Cumin)... 58
Jostaberry 58
Juniper Berries 58
Kaki (Persimmon) 58
Kale... 58
Kefir 58
Kelp (Large Seaweeds, Algae)....................................... 58
Kelp, Seaweed, Algae 59
Khorasan Wheat 59
Kiwi Fruit... 59
Kohlrabi 59
Kombu Seaweed.. 59
Lactose (Milk Sugar) 59
Ladyfinger Banana 59
Lamb (Organic, Freshly Cooked).................................. 59
Lamb's Lettuce, Corn Salad 60
Langouste... 60

Lard 60
Laurel, Bay Laurel, Sweet Bay, Bay Tree, True Laurel,
Grecian Laurel 60
Leek 60
Lemon 60
Lemon Peel, Lemon Zest 60
Lemonade 60
Lentils 61
Lettuce Iceberg 61
Lettuce: Head and Leaf Lettuces 61
Lime 61
Lime Blossom Tea, Limeflower, Flowers of Large-Leaved
Limetree 61
Lingonberry 61
Liquor, Clear 61
Liquor, Schnapps, Spirits, Cloudy (Not Colourless) 62
Liquorice Root 62
Lobster 62
Loganberry 62
Lychee 62
Macadamia 62
Malt Extract 63
Malt, Barley Malt 63
Maltodextrin 63
Maltose, Malt Sugar (Pure) 63
Mandarin Orange 63
Mango 63
Maple Syrup 63

Margarine 64
Marrow 64
Mascarpone Cheese... 64
Mate Tea... 64
Meat Extract 64
Meat. General 64
Melons (Except Watermelon)................................... 65
Meridian Fennel.. 65
Milk, Lactose-free 65
Milk, Pasteurised 65
Milk, UHT 65
Milk powder 65
Millet 66
Minced Meat (If Eaten Immediately After Its Production) 66
Minced Meat (Open Sale or Pre-Packed)................... 66
Mineral water, still 66
Mint 66
Mold cheeses, mould cheeses 66
Morel 67
Morello cherries 67
Mozzarella cheese 67
Mulberry 67
Mungbeans (germinated, sprouting) 67
Mushrooms, different types 67
Mustard, mustard seeds, mustardseed powder 67
Napa cabbage 68
Nashi pear 68
Nectarine 68

Nigella sativa oil 68
Nigella sativa seed 68
Nori seaweed 68
Nut grass 68
Nutmeg 69
Nutmeg flower 69
Nutmeg flower oil 69
Nuts 69
Oat drink, oat milk 69
Oats 69
Olive oil 70
Olives 70
Onion 70
Orange 70
Orange juice 70
Orange peel, orange zest 71
Oregano 71
Ostrich 71
Ostrich (organic, freshly cooked) 71
Oyster 71
Pak choi 71
Palm kernel oil 71
Palm oil, dendê oil 71
Palm sugar 72
Papaya, pawpaw 72
Paprika, hot 72
Paprika, sweet 72
Parsley 72

Parsnip 72
Passionfruit 72
Pasta (search individual ingredients, eg wheat, corn) 72
Paw paw 73
Peach 73
Peanuts.. 73
Pear 73
Pear, peeled canned in sugar syrup 73
Pearl sago 73
Peas (green) 74
Pea shoots 74
Pepper, black 74
Pepper, white 74
Peppermint tea 74
Perennial wall-rocket 74
Persian cumin 74
Persimmon 74
Pickled cabbage 75
Pickled cucumber 75
Pickled gherkin 75
Pickled vegetables 75
Pine nuts 75
Pineapple 75
Pistachio 75
Pitaya, pitahaya, dragon fruit 76
Pizza base (search individual ingredients, eg wheat, corn) . 76
Plaice 76
Plantains 76

Plum 76
Pomegranate juice 76
Popcorn (plain, popped) 76
Poppyseed 77
Porcini mushrooms 77
Pork 77
Pork (organic, freshly cooked) 77
Portabello mushrooms 77
Potato 77
Potato flour 77
Potato starch 78
Prunes 78
Pumpkin 78
Quail 78
Quince 78
Quinoa 78
Quinoa flakes 78
Rabbit 78
Radicchio 79
Radish 79
Raisins 79
Rapeseed oil 79
Raspberries 79
Red cabbage 79
Red onions 79
Red pepper, bell pepper 79
Redcurrants 80
Reindeer 80

Rice 80
Rice bran oil 80
Rice cakes 80
Rice flour 80
Rice milk 80
Rice noodles 81
Rice paper 81
Rice vinegar 81
Rosemary 81
Rutabaga, swede 81
Rye 81
Safflower oil 81
Saffron 82
Sage 82
Salmon 82
Sardines 82
Sauerkraut 82
Scallop 82
Sea bass 82
Sea bream 82
Seafood (fresh, unprocessed) 83
Seaweed 83
Sesame oil 83
Sesame seeds 83
Shallots 83
Sheep 83
Shiitake mushrooms 83
Shrimp 84

Skimmed milk 84
Sloe berries 84
Smoked fish (plain, no additives) 84
Smoked meat (plain, no additives) 84
Soba noodles 84
Sorbet 84
Sorghum 85
Sorghum flour 85
Soy sauce 85
Spaghetti squash 85
Spinach 86
Split peas 86
Squash (all varieties) 86
Star anise 86
Stevia 86
Strawberries 86
Sugar (white, brown, confectioner's) 86
Sunflower oil 86
Sunflower seeds 87
Sweet potatoes 87
Swiss chard 87
Tangerines 87
Tapioca 87
Tarragon 87
Tea 87
Thyme 88
Tofu 88
Tomatillos 88

Tomatoes 88
Trout 88
Tuna (fresh) 88
Turkey (fresh, unprocessed) 89
Turmeric 89
Turnips 89
Vanilla extract 89
Venison 89
Vinegar (distilled white, balsamic, wine, apple cider, but
not malt) 89
Walnuts 90
Watercress 90
Wheat 90
Wheatgrass.. 90
Whitefish 90
Wild rice 90
Wine 91
Xanthan gum... 91
Yams 91
Yogurt (plain, unflavored) 91
Zucchini 91

Introduction

Hi, and welcome to this book on following the gluten-free diet. I truly hope it helps, and I know how much it is needed. Trust me, I've made every mistake it's possible to make on the gluten-free diet! It can be an absolute minefield, but after well over a decade of living completely gluten-free, I can finally say I've made most of the mistakes (hopefully) and I don't accidentally gluten myself any more.

This book has been a passion project to put together. It's something I have needed and wanted myself for many years. I have had my battles with food intolerances and sensitivities, with gluten affecting my gut the worst. It was the very first thing I eliminated from my diet, and I have never gone back.

As well as all the painstaking research that has gone into this book, that means on a personal level I now know the potential stumbling blocks - the things that most books don't tell you; sauces with hidden gluten in them, fries that are listed as gluten-free on a menu but cooked in the same oil as a million other gluten-containing items, and simple human error. I can look after my own diet just fine these days, but only last week I was in a restaurant and served a burger (with no bun). It was only after taking a mouthful that I thought to double-check that the meat had no gluten in it... which is something over the years I've learnt is always a good idea. Of course it *did contain gluten*. How could I have forgotten to ask? (Incidentally, the server took precisely 9 dollars off the bill, which seemed a little low given that she'd just given me five days of stomach ache).

These are regular frustrations that we have to deal with, and I've seen far too many times over the years. It is why I have taken the initiative and got going with this book. It is, hopefully, the most reliable list of gluten-free books around, drawing from the best and most trusted gluten sources around. Here's how I approached this task.

- Step 1: lived gluten-free myself for more than a decade
- Step 2: made every mistake it is possible to make when it came to cooking, choosing, and ordering food.
- Step 3: found the most trusted sources for gluten-free content in food and realized a lot of them don't necessarily tell the whole story, or have omissions, or just don't provide the information in an easy-to-use way.
- Step 4: put this guide together.

So what actually is gluten?

Gluten is a group of proteins found in wheat, barley, and rye, and it hides in an incredible amount of food and drink products. You could call it the glue (which is a nice analogy) that helps food keep its shape. For some of us though, gluten wreaks havoc. It can cause many problems from digestive issues (my particular problem) to inflammation to severe autoimmune reactions.

Often gluten-containing foods can be tough to spot, so take this book wherever you go. And particularly in restaurants, in my experience it's worth checking, and checking again with your server on the gluten free content in food. Mistakes happen. I've been offered apologies, vouchers, free meals and all sorts after such mistakes. And I still ordered that gluten burger last week! It's a minefield. I hope this guide and a healthy dose of vigilance will help you avoid the same issues.

How to Use this Food List

This book is your gluten-free dictionary. It's got an alphabetized list of foods, drinks, and ingredients you can read through (if you really want) or simply search for any food, whenever you like.

I've sifted through the world's best resources and boiled down all that information into a simple rating system. Each item gets a score from 0 to 2, based on its gluten content.

Here's the breakdown:

0 - Generally safe. These foods should be gluten-free and safe on the gluten-free diet. (Though still check labels, be aware of cross contamination and potential errors)

1 - Extreme caution. There is debate around these foods, or they sometimes contain gluten. Proceed with caution.

2 - Avoid. Contains gluten and best avoided.

This means a score of 0 is good, and a score of 2 is - obviously - a red flag and very likely to contain gluten. Over time, with guidance from your practitioner, you can figure out which foods are safe and which ones to avoid.

Legal definitions of 'gluten-free'.

By law, in the U.S. and in many other countries, a food product can only be labeled "gluten-free" if it contains less than 20 parts per million (ppm) of gluten.

Now, you're possibly thinking, "Hang on, that means there's still gluten in there!" And you'd be absolutely right. Let's put this into context with an example. Picture this: if you took one million grains of rice, and only 20 of those grains were gluten, that's the equivalent of 20ppm. It's a tiny amount, but it's not zero.

So, even when a product says "gluten-free" on the label, it does quite often contain minute traces of gluten. I have a problem with this. If you're particularly sensitive to gluten or have been diagnosed with celiac disease, this can potentially be an issue. I've come across plenty of people for whom this is an issue, and indeed I think all of us who are gluten-free should be mindful of it.

Er, the Beers are (not) on me.

For example: Some beers are labeled "gluten-removed" or "gluten-reduced." These are made with traditional gluten-containing grains, but an enzyme is added during the brewing process that breaks down the gluten. These beers might meet the legal definition of "gluten-free" in that they contain less than 20ppm of gluten, but there's still debate in the medical community about whether these are safe for people with celiac disease or severe gluten intolerance. Everyone is different, but I would encourage you to avoid these unless your intolerance is very mild. You can find reliable beers

There are thankfully, reliably 100% gluten-free beers and alcohols. For example, Ghostfish Brewing Company out of Seattle have won multiple awards for their beers. They are produced in a dedicated brewery, made from gluten-free grains and are celiac safe.

Spirits such as vodka, gin, or whiskey are another area where confusion can arise. These spirits are often distilled from grains and the distillation process should technically remove all gluten proteins.

But there can be traces of gluten present due to potential cross-contamination in the manufacturing process. So, a vodka or a whiskey could potentially contain up to 20ppm of gluten, even if it's labeled as "gluten-free." It all depends on the brand, and what has been used to create the alcohol.

Crazy really, isn't it? Up to 20ppm of gluten is clearly not gluten-free but that is how it can be labeled.

I hope this section helps you. Everyone's sensitivity to gluten is different, and what works for one person might not work for another. You might be perfectly comfortable with the legal definition of 'gluten-free', or you might want a round 0ppm of gluten in your food. Discuss with your healthcare provider.

Sources

These excellent sources come highly recommended in your further research on gluten. I consider these to be the best gluten-free sources out there and in over a decade of being gluten-free myself have come to trust them. Check them out.

1. Celiac Disease Foundation (https://celiac.org): Lots of information about celiac disease and gluten-free living. Provides lists of foods and ingredients to avoid and those that are safe to eat.

2. Gluten-Free Living (https://www.glutenfreeliving.com): Practical advice, recipes, and tips for living gluten-free.

3. National Celiac Association (https://nationalceliac.org): Does what it says on the tin. Advice for understanding and managing celiac disease and gluten sensitivities.

4. [Gluten Intolerance Group](https://gluten.org): A leading source of consumer and industry information on gluten-free standards and labeling.

5. Beyond Celiac (https://www.beyondceliac.org): You'll guess from the name - this organization is a big help.

6. The Gluten-Free Society (https://www.glutenfreesociety.org): Highly respected and helpful.

7. Coeliac UK (https://www.coeliac.org.uk): Some UK based info, and some which is relevant for everyone on gluten-free foods, recipes, and tips.

8. [Verywell Fit](https://www.verywellfit.com): Not specifically gluten-free, provides information on lots of different diets including gluten-free.

9. Mayo Clinic (https://www.mayoclinic.org): Well known site with extensive resources on celiac disease and diets free of gluten.

10. American Dietetic Association (https://www.eatright.org): Helpful for knowing what to avoid, how to read labels, and so on.

Disclaimer

You must consult with your doctor, nutritionist, dietitian or healthcare provider before changing your diet. They have the expertise required to offer you personalized treatment.

Please remember this: The information contained in this book has been compiled from sources deemed reliable, and it is accurate to the best of our knowledge based on the respected sources above; however, the accuracy cannot be guaranteed and we cannot be held liable for any errors or omissions, or for any gluten contamination. Always check and double-check labels, ask servers, and consult the sources in this book.

Now, let's move on to the food list.

The Food List

Acerola - 0

Acerola is gluten-free.

Agave syrup - 0

Agave syrup is derived from a plant and is fine for those following a gluten-free diet.

Alcohol - 2

This is definitely one to be very mindful of. Some alcohols are gluten-free. See individual alcohols for details. Owing to the distillation process there is often significant amounts of gluten in alcohol and so this is too broad to score anything else but 2. Check individual alcohols for more details and be mindful of how legal definitions of gluten may not be 0ppm (see intro for more on this).

Algae and algae derivatives - 0

Algae is plant-based. It is gluten-free.

Almond - 0

Almonds should be gluten-free and almond flour is one of our favorite gluten-free flours to bake with. Remember, unlike wheat flour, gluten-free flours lack gluten, which provides elasticity and structure to baked goods. To mimic these properties, a blend of different gluten-free flours and starches can be used, including almond. Xanthan gum or guar gum can be added as a gluten substitute to provide the necessary elasticity. Experiment with different combinations to find the perfect blend. It's a process, for sure. I quite like combining almond with coconut. Each individual flour doesn't quite work on its own, but together is a nice blend.

Amaranth - 0

Amaranth is useful; a gluten-free grain.

Anchovies - 0

Anchovy is gluten-free. However, if store-bought or canned, some preparations or brands may contain gluten in sauces.

Anise, aniseed - 0

Anise should be fine for those following gluten-free.

Apple - 0

Apples are fine - naturally gluten-free.

Apple cider vinegar - 0

Apple cider vinegar is made from apples. It's gluten-free. I can't think of any scenario where gluten would be added to ACV, but check the label.

Apricot - 0

Commonly gluten-free.

Artichoke - 0

Artichokes are fine on the GF diet.

Artificial sweeteners - 1

Many artificial sweeteners are gluten-free, but some may contain gluten due to additives. Amazing really that this should be the case.

Asimina triloba - 0

More commonly known as pawpaw, it is commonly gluten-free.

Asparagus - 0

Asparagus is gluten-free.

Aubergine - 0

Also known as eggplant, aubergines are fine - gluten-free.

Avocado - 0

Avocados are completely gluten-free, and a great source of healthy fats.

Bamboo shoots - 0

Bamboo shoots are gluten-free

Banana - 0

Barbary fig - 0

Also known as prickly pear, and fine for those who are gluten-free.

Barley - 2

Avoid. Barley is a gluten-containing grain and should be avoided. It is sometimes labeled separately to gluten on products so be mindful of this.

Barley malt, malt - 2

Barley malt and malt are derived from barley, the gluten-containing grain mentioned above. These should be avoided. Watch for labeling.

Basil - 0

Bay laurel, laurel - 0

Bay laurel is a plant and is normally gluten-free.

Beans (pulses) - 0

Beans should be completely gluten-free. However, cross-contamination can occur in processing facilities, so always check labels.

Beef (depending on age of beef, organic, freshly cooked) - 1

While beef is gluten-free, processed or flavored beef products may contain gluten. Always check labels.

Beer - 2

Most beer is made from malted barley and contains gluten, although gluten-free beers are now available. See the introduction for more.

That means beer scores a 2, however some beer-makers and breweries work in dedicated facilities. They use gluten-free grains and are celiac safe.

Beetroot - 0

This root vegetable is gluten-free, but watch out for beetroot sold in salads or sauces.

Bell pepper (hot) - 0

Bell pepper (sweet) - 0

Bison (organic, freshly cooked) - 0

Inherently gluten-free, provided it is fresh and cooked without gluten-containing additives.

Bivalves (mussels, oyster, clams, scallops) - 0

Be aware of sauces and preparation methods that may introduce gluten.

Black caraway - 0

Black caraway is a spice and gluten-free.

Black caraway oil - 0

The oil derived from black caraway is also gluten-free.

Blackberry - 0

Blackcurrants - 0

Blue cheeses, mold cheeses - 1

These cheeses just might contain gluten due to cross-contamination in the aging process.

Blue fenugreek - 0

Blueberries - 0

Absolutely fine.

Bok choi - 0

Borlotti beans - 0

Check for cross-contamination in processing.

Bouillon (yeast extract / meat extract / glutamate) - 2

Many bouillon cubes and powders contain gluten in the form of wheat flour or wheat starch, or through additives. Check very, very carefully!

Boysenberry - 0

Boysenberries are gluten-free - no problem.

Brandy - 2

Brandy is a distilled alcohol that can potentially contain gluten due to distillation from gluten grains. If you are a brandy drinker, you could contact your favorite brand for more details as each brand varies.

Brazil nut - 0

Gluten free, but check for cross-contamination in processing.

Bread - 2

Most bread is made from wheat flour and thus contains gluten, but gluten-free breads are available.

Broad bean - 0

Broad beans are gluten-free, as area all beans.

Broad-leaved garlic - 0

This herb is gluten-free.

Broccoli - 0

Completely gluten-free.

Brown algae, algae - 0

Always a good idea to check the labels for added gluten in any form, but this is gluten-free.

Brussels sprouts - 0

A Christmas favorite. Brussels sprouts are gluten-free, but are often prepared on festive occasions with sauces and glazes.

Buckrams - 0

This plant is completely gluten-free.

Buckwheat - 0

Despite its name, buckwheat is not a type of wheat and is gluten-free, but check for cross-contamination in processing.

Butter - 1

Butter is gluten-free, but flavored or spreadable versions may contain gluten. In addition, in our family there are regular arguments about the butter dish containing little crumbs from some gluten-containing toast!

Butterkaese - 0

Butterkaese is a type of cheese and is generally gluten-free, but check labels to be sure.

Buttermilk - 0

Buttermilk is probably gluten-free, but check labels to ensure no gluten-containing additives are included.

Cabbage, green or white - 0

Cabbage is always gluten-free.

Cactus pear - 0

Cactus pear, also known as prickly pear, is always gluten-free.

Caraway - 0

Caraway seeds are probably gluten-free.

Cardamom - 0

This spice is gluten-free.

Carrot - 0

Carrots are gluten-free.

Cashew nut - 0

Cashews are gluten-free, but check for cross-contamination in processing.

Cassava - 0

Cassava is a root vegetable that is comes out of the soil gluten-free. It's a great gluten-free flour alternative which I love to cook with.

Cassava flour - 0

Cassava flour is made from the gluten-free cassava root. See above - one of my favourite gluten free flours.

Cauliflower - 0

Another veg, gluten-free.

Celery - 0

Celery is gluten-free.

Celery cabbage - 0

This vegetable is gluten-free.

Cep - 0

Cep is a type of mushroom, no gluten.

Chamomile tea - 0

Pure chamomile tea is fine, but check labels as some flavored or blended teas may contain gluten.

Champagne - 2

Champagne is a type of wine, and while the grapes are gluten-free, the fining process can introduce trace amounts of gluten. Which is something I didn't know. Check with your supplier.

Chard stalks - 0

Chard is a type of vegetable - fine.

Chayote - 0

Chayote is a type of squash that contains no gluten.

Cheddar cheese - 0

Cheddar cheese is typically gluten-free, but some brands may introduce gluten during processing, so always check the label.

Cheese made from unpasteurised "raw" milk - 0

Cheese made from raw milk tends to be gluten-free, but it is always a good idea to check the labels for any added ingredients that may contain gluten.

Cheese: soft cheeses - 0

Soft cheeses are typically gluten-free. As with any cheese, it is always best to check the label for any gluten-containing additives.

Cheese: hard cheese, all well matured cheeses - 0

Hard, well-matured cheeses should be gluten-free, but again, always check the label for any gluten-containing additives.

Cherry - 0

Cherries are gluten-free. Simple.

Chestnut, sweet chestnut - 0

Chestnuts are gluten-free.

Chia - 0

Chia seeds are on their own, gluten-free.

Chicken - 0

Chicken is naturally gluten-free, provided it is cooked without any gluten-containing additives. As noted above, cooked chicken often contains gluten either in a glaze or in the chicken itself.

This may seem trivial, but it's really worth looking out for. Look for cooked chicken ingredients in shops, and products such as chicken liver paté which often contains gluten.

Chickpeas - 0

Chickpeas are gluten-free.

Chicory - 0

Chicory is gluten-free.

Chili pepper, red, fresh - 0

Fresh red chili peppers are gluten-free.

Chives - 0

Chives are gluten-free and should be safe for celiacs or anyone with gluten sensitivity.

Chocolate - 1

Some chocolate, especially milk and white chocolate, can contain gluten due to additives or cross-contamination during production. Some cheaper chocolate brands 'fill out' their chocolate with gluten-containing ingredients. Even expensive brands sometimes manage to somehow sneak some gluten in (why!). Check individual brands.

Cilantro - 0

Cilantro, also known as coriander in some places, is gluten-free.

Cinnamon - 0

Cinnamon is gluten-free.

Citrus fruits - 0

Citrus fruits, including oranges, lemons, limes, and grapefruits, are gluten-free.

Clover - 0

Clover is naturally gluten-free.

Cloves - 0

Cloves are always gluten-free.

Cocoa butter - 0

Cocoa butter is gluten-free.

Cocoa drinks - 1

Cocoa drinks can sometimes contain gluten due to additives or cross-contamination in production, so always check the label.

Cocoa, cocoa powder (chocolate, etc.) - 0

Pure cocoa and cocoa powder are gluten-free, but always check labels as some brands may add gluten-containing additives.

Coconut fat, coconut oil - 0

Coconut fat and coconut oil contain no gluten.

Coconut, coconut shavings, coconut milk - 0

Coconuts, coconut shavings, and coconut milk are all gluten-free.

Coconut is a good gluten-free flour to bake with. Unlike wheat flour, gluten-free flours lack gluten (obviously), which provides elasticity and structure to baking. So we need to find something to replace it. Coconut flour on its own can be quite dry. Try combining rice flour, almond flour, and coconut flour, each bringing unique flavors and textures, and providing a similar consistency too.

Coffee - 0

Everybody asks about coffee. The good news is; plain coffee - beans or ground - is just that, coffee, and gluten-free. However flavored coffees may contain gluten or be cross-contaminated. Powdered creamer may contain gluten.

Cola-drinks - 1

Cola drinks are a gray area. They may contain barley malt, which can occasionally contain gluten. It's always best to check the label. In addition, look out for the caramel coloring ingredient which could also contain gluten.

Common sea-buckthorn - 0

Sea-buckthorn is gluten-free.

Coriander - 0

Coriander is fine.

Corn - 0

Corn is gluten-free, but one to look out for. Beware of cross-contamination, especially when eating out or eating processed foods. Watch out for products like 'cornflakes' - yes, of course, it would be reasonable to think cornflakes are only made of corn, but that's not necessarily the case. It's a mistake I've made before, see below.

Corn salad, lamb's lettuce - 0

Corn salad, also known as lamb's lettuce, is gluten-free according to my sources.

Cornflakes (if no additives) - 1

Plain cornflakes would be typically gluten-free, but many brands add malt flavoring or other additives that contain gluten. Always check the label. For example, Kellogg's Corn Flakes have gluten in them. Even though the main ingredient is milled corn, the cereal also contains barley malt extract, which has gluten in it.

Courgette - 0

Courgette, also known as zucchini, is fine. Often used in gluten-free baking.

Cowberry - 0

Cowberries, also known as lingonberries, are ordinarily gluten-free.

Crab - 0

Crab is gluten-free, but beware of sauces and preparation methods that may introduce gluten.

Cranberry - 0

Cranberries are fine.

Cranberry nectar - 0

Cranberry nectar is gluten-free according to my sources., but always check the label for any gluten-containing additives.

Crawfish - 0

Crawfish, also known as crayfish, are gluten-free, but beware of sauces and preparation methods that may introduce gluten.

Cream cheeses (means: very young cheeses), plain, without additives - 0

Cream cheeses are generally gluten-free, but flavored or spreadable versions may contain gluten.

Cream, sweet, without additives - 0

Sweet cream without additives is gluten-free.

Cress: garden cress - 0

Garden cress is generally gluten-free, unless contaminated in some way.

Cucumber - 0

Cucumbers are ordinarily gluten-free.

Cumin - 0

Cumin does not contain gluten. Check the label though.

Curd cheese - 0

Curd cheese is typically gluten-free, but check labels to be sure.

Curry - 1

Curry is a blend of spices, all of which *should* be gluten-free. However, often there will be some sort of gluten-containing ingredient in there, so check carefully. Also be aware of contamination during processing.

Dates (dried, desiccated) - 0

Dates are generally gluten-free, but check labels to ensure no gluten-containing additives or cross-contamination.

Dextrose - 0

Dextrose, a type of sugar, is gluten-free according to my sources.

Dill - 0

Dill is normally gluten-free.

Distilled white vinegar - 0

Distilled white vinegar is typically gluten-free. Vinegar made from gluten grains can be a source of gluten, but the distillation process should remove any gluten.

Dog rose - 0

Dog rose, a type of wild rose, is gluten-free.

Dragon fruit, pitaya - 0

Dragon fruit, also known as pitaya, is fine.

Dried meat (any kind) - 1

Definitely watch out. Dried meats can sometimes contain gluten due to additives or flavorings, so always check the label.

Dry-cured ham - 0

Dry-cured ham is typically gluten-free but not always, so check labels.

Duck - 0

Duck is fine - gluten-free, provided it is prepared and cooked without gluten-containing ingredients.

Earth almond - 0

Earth almonds, also known as tiger nuts, are no problem on the gluten-free diet.

Egg white - 0

Egg whites are gluten-free.

Egg yolk - 0

Egg yolks are gluten-free - they're just eggs.

Eggplant - 0

Eggplant, also known as aubergine, is gluten-free.

Eggs, chicken egg, whole egg - 0

Eggs are gluten-free. Any egg in the diet of the hen is broken down in the digestive process, meaning there will be no gluten in your egg.

Elderflower cordial - 1

Elderflower cordial can

Elderflower cordial - 1

Elderflower cordial can sometimes contain gluten due to additives or processing methods. Always check the label to be sure.

Endive - 0

Endive is gluten-free.

Energy drinks - 1

Many energy drinks can contain gluten due to added ingredients or cross-contamination during manufacturing. Always check labels.

Entrails - 0

Entrails, or offal, from animals are gluten-free, but you do need to be aware of how they are prepared and cooked, as there could well be gluten in this process.

Espresso - 0

Your morning espresso is fine, but flavored espressos and additives may contain gluten.

Ethanol - 1

Ethanol itself is usually gluten-free, but be cautious as it can be derived from gluten-containing grains and a small amount of gluten may be present.

Ewe's milk, sheep's milk - 0

Sheep's milk is gluten-free.

Extract of malt - 2

Malt extract is typically made from barley, a gluten-containing grain, so it is not safe for those with celiac disease or gluten intolerance.

Farmer's cheese (a type of fresh cheese) - 0

Farmer's cheese is typically gluten-free, but check labels to be sure.

Fennel - 0

Fennel is generally gluten-free.

Fennel flower (Nigella sativa) - 0

Fennel flower is gluten-free.

Fennel flower oil (Nigella sativa) - 0

Fennel flower oil is also fine.

Fenugreek - 0

Fenugreek is gluten-free.

Feta cheese - 0

Feta cheese is typically gluten-free, but check labels to be sure.

Figs (fresh or dried) - 0

Figs are gluten-free.

Fish (freshly caught within an hour or frozen within an hour) - 0

Fish on its own is gluten-free, provided it is not prepared with gluten-containing ingredients.

Fish (in the shop in the cooling rack or on ice) - 0

Fish from a store should also be gluten-free, but always check for any added ingredients, especially in pre-seasoned or marinated varieties.

Flaxseed (linseed) - 0

Flaxseed is gluten-free, but as with all seeds, it's best to look for versions labeled gluten-free to avoid cross-contamination.

Fontina cheese - 0

Fontina cheese is typically gluten-free, but check labels to be sure.

Fries, chips - 1

In theory, if potato fries are made from one ingredient (potatoes) then they are gluten-free. But in practice fries are often a) coated with a gluten-containing ingredient or b) cooked in oil which has already cooked lots of other gluten-containing foods. Be extremely cautious and ask restaurants if they have a separate fryer for fries which is gluten-free.

Fructose (fruit sugar) - 0

Fructose, or fruit sugar, is naturally gluten-free.

Game - 0

Game meat, like venison or quail, is naturally gluten-free, provided it's not prepared with gluten-containing ingredients. (Dried game in the form of jerky or bars may well contain gluten)

Garden cress - 0

Garden cress is gluten-free.

Garlic (usually well tolerated) - 0

Garlic is gluten-free.

Geheimratskaese, Geheimrats cheese - 0

Geheimratskaese, or Geheimrat cheese, is typically gluten-free, but check labels to be sure.

German turnip - 0

German turnip, also known as kohlrabi, is gluten-free.

Ginger - 0

Ginger is gluten-free.

Glucose - 0

Glucose, a type of sugar, is gluten-free, but watch out for other ingredients.

Goat's milk, goat milk - 0

Goat's milk is gluten-free.

Goji berry, Chinese wolfberry, Chinese boxthorn, Himalayan goji, Tibetan goji - 0

These berries are gluten-free.

Goose (organic, freshly cooked) - 0

Goose is gluten-free, provided it is prepared and cooked without gluten-containing ingredients.

Gooseberry, gooseberries - 0

Gooseberries are just berries, and gluten-free.

Gouda cheese (young) - 0

Young Gouda cheese is typically gluten-free, but check labels to be sure.

Gouda cheese, old - 0

Old Gouda cheese is also typically fine.

Gourds - 0

Gourds, like pumpkins and squash, are yes, gluten-free.

Grapefruit - 0

Grapefruit is gluten-free.

Grapes - 0

Grapes are gluten-free.

Gravy - 1

Gravy, especially in restaurants and ready-made versions, often contains flour as a thickening agent, which contains gluten. It's of course possible to make gluten-free gravy using alternatives like cornstarch or gluten-free flour mixes, but don't rely on store-bought or restaurant gravy unless you can get assurances.. Always check labels if buying from the store, and inquire at restaurants.

Green algae, algae - 0

Green algae is fine, gluten-free.

Green beans - 0

Green beans are gluten-free, but as always, what are they cooked in?

Green peas - 0

Fine. Green peas are gluten-free.

Green split peas - 0

Green split peas are also gluten-free.

Green tea - 0

Green tea is absolutely gluten-free as long as it is just tea, but flavored or blended varieties may contain gluten, so check labels.

Guava - 0

Guava is gluten-free. In addition, canned guava should be fine too.

Ham (dried, cured) - 1

Dried, cured ham can sometimes contain gluten due to flavorings or additives. You'd be surprised at how often this occurs... so always check the label or ask your butcher.

Hazelnut - 0

This nut is gluten-free.

Hemp seeds (Cannabis sativa) - 0

Hemp seeds are fine.

Herbal teas with medicinal herbs - 1

Seems crazy, but herbal teas can sometimes contain gluten due to cross-contamination during processing or from added flavors. Check labels.

Honey - 0

Honey is gluten-free.

Horseradish - 0

Horseradish is gluten-free, although horseradish sauce may not be. If in a restaurant, ask to see the label, or avoid.

Hot chocolate - 1

Hot chocolate can contain gluten, especially if it's pre-packaged or from a mix. Always check labels. (Do I sound like a broken record?!)

Indian fig opuntia, Barbary fig, cactus pear, spineless cactus, prickly pear, tuna - 0

These types of cactus fruits are all naturally gluten-free.

Innards - 1

Innards, or offal, from animals are gluten-free, but be aware of how they are prepared and cooked. Often they could be prepared with some sort of grain, hence the caution here.

Inverted sugar syrup - 0

Inverted sugar syrup is gluten-free.

Ispaghula, psyllium seed husks - 0

Ispaghula, also known as psyllium seed husks, is gluten-free.

Jeera (Cumin) - 0

Jeera, also known as cumin, is suitable for the GF diet. For extra safety, buy spices that are sold as a single ingredient spice, rather than a mix.

Jostaberry - 0

Jostaberry - yes, gluten-free.

Juniper Berries - 0

Juniper berries - fine, these are gluten-free.

Kaki (Persimmon) - 0

Kaki, or Persimmon, is fine for the gluten-free diet.

Kale - 0

Kale is a leafy green vegetable that is gluten-free.

Kefir - 0

Kefir is generally gluten-free, but check labels for potential added ingredients. Some store bought products may use non-gluten-free oats or other products containing gluten to add flavor or texture.

Kelp (Large Seaweeds, Algae) - 0

Kelp, a type of large seaweed or algae, is typically gluten-free.

Kelp, Seaweed, Algae - 0

These are different types of sea vegetables and are suitable for the gluten-free diet.

Khorasan Wheat - 2

Contains gluten. Avoid.

Kiwi Fruit - 0

Fine. A good gluten-free snack option.

Kohlrabi - 0

Guten-free.

Kombu Seaweed - 0

This seaweed is typically gluten-free.

Lactose (Milk Sugar) - 0

Lactose is a type of sugar found in milk and should be fine, gluten-free.

Ladyfinger Banana - 0

Ladyfinger bananas, like all bananas, are gluten-free. Bananas may well be your gluten-free baking friend, too.

Lamb (Organic, Freshly Cooked) - 0

Freshly cooked, organic lamb is gluten-free on its own, of course. However be cautious of any seasonings or marinades used.

Lamb's Lettuce, Corn Salad - 0

Both lamb's lettuce and corn salad are also gluten-free.

Langouste - 0

Langouste is gluten-free but often comes with a sauce - check.

Lard - 0

Lard, a type of fat, is gluten-free.

Laurel, Bay Laurel, Sweet Bay, Bay Tree, True Laurel, Grecian Laurel - 0

Gluten free, typically

Leek - 0

Leeks are a type of vegetable and are ordinarily gluten-free, unless cooked in a sauce (often served in a white or creamy sauce so check).

Lemon - 0

Lemons are fine.

Lemon Peel, Lemon Zest - 0

Also fine.

Lemonade - 1

While lemons are gluten-free, some commercially-prepared lemonades may contain gluten (I know, how!?) so check labels carefully.

Lentils - 0

Lentils are naturally gluten-free. However, they may be cross-contaminated during processing, so ensure they are labeled gluten-free.

Lettuce Iceberg - 0

Iceberg lettuce, like all types of lettuce, is typically gluten-free.

Lettuce: Head and Leaf Lettuces - 0

Lettuce is fine. Side note: Watch out for double dippers at buffets when loading your plate with delicious lettuce and other salads - especially if it's right next to the pasta. A bit of gluten double-dipping is not welcome.

Lime - 0

Limes, like all fruits, are fine.

Lime Blossom Tea, Limeflower, Flowers of Large-Leaved Limetree - 0

Lime blossom tea and lime flowers are gluten-free.

Lingonberry - 0

No probs.

Liquor, Clear - 1

One to be very cautious on. Clear liquors can vary greatly in their gluten content. It really depends on the distillation process, and sometimes the ingredients too. Some are made from grains that contain gluten, so check labels carefully. You may need to do some sleuthing on your favorite liquors. Liquors that use potatoes in the distillation process may end up being your friend.

Liquor, Schnapps, Spirits, Cloudy (Not Colourless) - 1

See above. Cloudy spirits and schnapps can contain gluten, especially if made from grains, so read labels carefully.

Liquorice Root - 0

Liquorice root itself is gluten-free, but processed liquorice sweets often contain gluten, so - yet again - check labels.

Lobster - 0

Lobster, like all shellfish, is gluten-free, but be aware of any potential sauces or seasonings.

Loganberry - 0

Fine.

Lychee - 0

Lychee is a fruit that is gluten-free. Lychee Martinis may not be - so check!

Macadamia - 0

Macadamia nuts are gluten-free.

Malt Extract - 2

A definite no-no. Malt extract is made from barley, which contains gluten.

Malt, Barley Malt - 2

Again, avoid. Malt, including barley malt, is made from barley, which contains gluten.

Maltodextrin - 1

Potentially avoid. Maltodextrin is a processed food ingredient. In the U.S., it is typically made from corn or potatoes and is gluten-free, but in Europe, it can be made from wheat, so check labels carefully.

Maltose, Malt Sugar (Pure) - 2

Definitely avoid. Maltose, also known as malt sugar, is made from barley, which contains gluten.

Mandarin Orange - 0

Oranges are fine.

Mango - 0

Mangoes are gluten-free.

Maple Syrup - 0

Pure maple syrup is probably gluten-free, but some brands may contain additives, so check labels.

Margarine - 1

While margarine is typically gluten-free, some brands may include additives or thickeners that contain gluten, so check labels carefully. Margarine can contain some surprising ingredients.

Marrow - 0

This is gluten-free.

Mascarpone Cheese - 0

Mascarpone cheese is gluten-free, but check labels to ensure no gluten-containing additives have been used.

Mate Tea - 0

Mate tea is made from the gluten-free yerba mate plant.

Meat Extract - 1

Meat extract can sometimes contain gluten due to added ingredients or flavorings, so always check the label. This is definitely one to be very cautious of.

Meat. General - 1

All meat should be gluten-free. But, (and it's a big but), processing, flavorings, or cross-contamination can introduce gluten. Cooked chicken in stores - for example - often has gluten injected into it to bulk it up (doesn't sound very appetizing does it.)

In addition, burgers often contain meat, so always, always ask your server (and see the personal story in the introduction for how you can sometimes have issues with burgers. Some chains are better than others for burgers, and at time of writing, Five Guys is a chain that has given us better information and options than many other chains.

Melons (Except Watermelon) - 0

Melons are suitable for gluten-free eaters.

Meridian Fennel - 0

Fine for non-gluten eaters.

Milk, Lactose-free - 0

Lactose-free milk is gluten-free, as indeed is all milk.

Milk, Pasteurised - 0

Pasteurised milk, like all milk, is gluten-free.

Milk, UHT - 0

Again, gluten-free...

Milk powder - 0

All milk products should be fine. Milk powder is made from milk, which is gluten-free. Unless anything is added, this should be fine.

Millet - 0

Millet is a type of grain that should be gluten-free, and very popular in the gluten-free community (yes, there is a community of us!)

Minced Meat (If Eaten Immediately After Its Production) - 0

Freshly minced meat is gluten-free, but be aware of any potential seasonings or additives. We like to get our meat minced fresh at the butchers.

Minced Meat (Open Sale or Pre-Packed) - 1

Pre-packaged minced meat can sometimes contain gluten due to added fillers or flavorings, so always check labels.

Mineral water, still - 0

Still mineral water is just that - water - and gluten-free. Same for sparkling.

Mint - 0

Mint in its natural form is gluten-free.

Mold cheeses, mould cheeses - 1

Some mold cheeses are made with cultures that could contain gluten, so always check labels. The website *Beyond Celiac* says; *'Some suggest that mold cultures of cheese may be grown on wheat or rye bread, so read the ingredients label.*

Generally, unless the ingredients label includes wheat, barley, rye or their derivatives, cheese should be safe.'

Morel - 0

Morel mushrooms are gluten-free.

Morello cherries - 0

Morello cherries are gluten-free in their natural state.

Mozzarella cheese - 0

Most mozzarella cheese is gluten-free but double-check for any additives on the label.

Mulberry - 0

Mulberries are typically gluten-free.

Mungbeans (germinated, sprouting) - 0

Mungbeans are gluten-free, even when germinated or sprouted.

Mushrooms, different types - 0

Mushrooms of all types are gluten-free, but often prepared with sauces, additives, other ingredients to be watchful for.

Mustard, mustard seeds, mustardseed powder - 1

Unfortunately, a lot of mustards contain gluten. Mustard, its seeds, and powder are gluten-free, but check packaged mustards for gluten, and also be wary of sauces containing mustard. Note - this is one ingredient that in our experience non-gluten intolerant 'normies' don't know much about, and as a result will proudly serve you something 'gluten-free', that has been cooked in a gluten-containing mustard sauce.

Napa cabbage - 0

Napa cabbage is generally gluten-free.

Nashi pear - 0

Nashi pears, like all pears, are inherently gluten-free.

Nectarine - 0

Yep, fine.

Nigella sativa oil - 0

Oil derived from Nigella sativa (black cumin) does not contain gluten.

Nigella sativa seed - 0

The seeds of Nigella sativa are gluten-free, as is the oil

Nori seaweed - 0

Nori seaweed is fine, gluten-free.

Nut grass - 0

Nut grass is a plant and does not contain gluten.

Nutmeg - 0

Nutmeg in its pure form is gluten-free.

Nutmeg flower - 0

The flower of the nutmeg plant does not contain gluten.

Nutmeg flower oil - 0

Oil derived from the flower of the nutmeg plant does not contain gluten.

Nuts - 0

Nuts in their natural, raw form are gluten-free. This includes pine nuts, pistachios, cashews, Brazil nuts, almonds, pecans, macadamia nuts, peanuts, walnuts, and other natural nuts. Be cautious with flavored nuts, which may contain gluten-containing additives. The same goes for pre-packaged nuts.

Oat drink, oat milk - 1

Oats themselves don't contain gluten, but are often contaminated with it. Check labels to ensure your oat milk is certified gluten-free.

Oats - 1

Always look for oats labeled 'gluten-free'. Oats don't tend to contain gluten but are often processed in facilities that also handle gluten-containing grains, leading to cross-contamination. In addition, many people with gluten sensitivity don't eat oats. This from the NHS website. *"Oats do not contain gluten, but many people with coeliac disease avoid eating them because they can become contaminated with other cereals that contain gluten."* Look for oats and oat products specifically labeled as gluten-free.

Oat flour is a good potential flour to bake with, but again, it must be specifically labeled gluten-free. Top tip: try combining oat flour with other flours such as almond, coconut, or rice flour.

Olive oil - 0

Pure olive oil is gluten-free.

Olives - 0

Olives are fine, but always check labels for any potential additives.

Onion - 0

Onions are gluten-free.

Orange - 0

Fruit is a great way for kids to enjoy sweet treats on a GF diet.

Orange juice - 0

Pure orange juice is gluten-free, but always check labels for additives.

Orange peel, orange zest - 0

Orange peel and zest are gluten-free.

Oregano - 0

Oregano in its natural form is gluten-free.

Ostrich - 0

Ostrich meat is gluten-free.

Ostrich (organic, freshly cooked) - 0

Freshly cooked organic ostrich is also gluten-free.

Oyster - 0

Oysters are gluten-free.

Pak choi - 0

Pak choi, or bok choy, is gluten-free.

Palm kernel oil - 0

Palm kernel oil is fine, gluten-free.

Palm oil, dendê oil - 0

Palm oil and dendê oil are gluten-free. Beware oil that has already been used to cook something else containing gluten, then used again.

Palm sugar - 0

Palm sugar is a natural sugar that does not contain gluten.

Papaya, pawpaw - 0

Both papaya and pawpaw are gluten-free.

Paprika, hot - 0

Hot paprika is inherently gluten-free. Watch out for additives in seasonings.

Paprika, sweet - 0

Sweet paprika is gluten-free. Watch out for additives in seasonings.

Parsley - 0

Parsley is fine, gluten-free.

Parsnip - 0

Parsnips are gluten-free veggies.

Passionfruit - 0

Passionfruit is gluten-free.

Pasta (search individual ingredients, eg wheat, corn) - 2

Traditional pasta is made from wheat and contains gluten. There are gluten-free pasta options available made from other grains like corn and rice and pea, but always check labels to confirm they're gluten-free. In restaurants ask for gluten-free pasta to be cooked in separate water in a separate pot (important - this does not always happen.)

Paw paw - 0

Paw paw, another name for papaya, is gluten-free.

Peach - 0

Peaches are gluten-free, and a great kids gluten-free snack.

Peanuts - 1

Peanuts are gluten-free, but be cautious with pre-packaged or flavored peanuts, which may contain gluten-containing additives. In fact this is quite often...so we have given it a score of 1.

Pear - 0

Pears are gluten-free.

Pear, peeled canned in sugar syrup - 1

Canned fruits can sometimes contain additives or be processed in facilities that handle gluten. Check labels to ensure they're gluten-free.

Pearl sago - 0

Pearl sago, a type of starch from certain palm stems, is gluten-free.

Peas (green) - 0

Green peas are consistently gluten-free.

Pea shoots - 0

Pea shoots, the young leaves of the pea plant, are also gluten-free.

Pepper, black - 0

Black pepper in its pure form is gluten-free.

Pepper, white - 0

White pepper is gluten-free.

Peppermint tea - 0

Peppermint tea is typically gluten-free, but always check labels to ensure there are no additives or flavorings that contain gluten.

Perennial wall-rocket - 0

Perennial wall-rocket, a type of herb, does not contain gluten.

Persian cumin - 0

Persian cumin, like all cumin, is gluten-free.

Persimmon - 0

Also, gluten-free.

Pickled cabbage - 1

While cabbage is gluten-free, pickling processes and additives can introduce gluten. Always check labels.

Pickled cucumber - 1

Similar to cabbage, cucumbers are inherently gluten-free, but the pickling process can introduce gluten. Check labels.

Pickled gherkin - 1

Gherkins are gluten-free, but the pickling process may introduce gluten. Check labels.

Pickled vegetables - 1

While vegetables are on their own gluten-free, the pickling process and potential additives can introduce gluten. Check labels.

Pine nuts - 0

Pine nuts are inherently gluten-free.

Pineapple - 0

Pineapple is gluten-free.

Pistachio - 0

Pistachios are normally gluten-free. Be careful of any seasoning.

Pitaya, pitahaya, dragon fruit - 0

All these names refer to the same fruit, which is gluten-free.

Pizza base (search individual ingredients, eg wheat, corn) - 2

Traditional pizza bases are made from wheat and therefore contain gluten. However, gluten-free alternatives are available and are usually made from grains like corn and rice. Always check labels to ensure they're gluten-free.

Plaice - 0

Plaice, a type of flatfish, is consistently gluten-free.

Plantains - 0

Similar to bananas, and are generally gluten-free.

Plum - 0

Pomegranate - 0

Pomegranate juice - 0

Similar to the above, pure pomegranate juice should be gluten-free, but always check labels to ensure there are no additives or flavorings that contain gluten.

Popcorn (plain, popped) - 1

Be careful with flavored popcorn, as it may contain gluten-containing additives. Plain popcorn with no additives that has been popped is gluten-free.

Poppyseed - 0

Porcini mushrooms - 0

Porcini mushrooms are gluten-free.

Pork - 1

Pork in its natural state is gluten-free. Processed pork products, such as sausages or bacon, as they may contain gluten. Sausages are a particular culprit here, and it's worth remembering this in restaurants too.

Pork (organic, freshly cooked) - 0

Freshly cooked organic pork with no additives or other ingredients is gluten-free.

Portabello mushrooms - 0

Potato - 0

Potatoes are generally gluten-free, and a great carb alternative when bread isn't an option. NB - a quick note on gnocchi - the delicious Italian potato dish. In a good restaurant, gnocchi will normally be gluten-free. However store-bought gnocchi often contains wheat or gluten.

Potato flour - 0

As above.

Potato starch - 0

And again - as above.

Prunes - 0

Dried plums, they are gluten-free.

Pumpkin - 0

Pumpkin seeds - 0

Quail - 0

Quail meat is gluten-free.

Quince - 0

Quinoa - 0

Quinoa is a gluten-free grain. However, it's a good idea to buy quinoa that is labeled gluten-free to avoid cross-contamination.

Quinoa flakes - 0

Like quinoa itself, quinoa flakes are gluten-free. Always check for gluten-free labeling to avoid potential cross-contamination.

Rabbit - 0

Radicchio - 0

Radicchio, a type of leaf chicory, is fine - yes, gluten-free.

Radish - 0

Raisins - 0

These are gluten-free.

Rapeseed oil - 0

Rapeseed oil on its own is fine, but check for any added ingredients.

Raspberries - 0

These berries are just that - berries, and nothing else... gluten-free.

Red cabbage - 0

Red cabbage is gluten-free.

Red onions - 0

Red onions, like all onions, are gluten-free.

Red pepper, bell pepper - 0

Peppers have been covered elsewhere. Red peppers or bell peppers are generally gluten-free.

Redcurrants - 0

Redcurrants are always gluten-free.

Reindeer - 0

A bit obscure perhaps. However reindeer meat is gluten-free.

Rice - 0

All types of rice (white, brown, basmati, jasmine, etc.) are gluten-free. Some experts and sites suggest avoiding rice from bulk bins at the grocery store to avoid cross-contamination.

Rice bran oil - 0

Rice bran oil, which is extracted from the outer layer of rice, is gluten-free according to my sources.

Rice cakes - 1

Rice cakes are typically gluten-free and in fact a handy and reliable gluten-free snack. Always check labels as they may contain additives or be processed in a facility that handles gluten.

Rice flour - 0

Rice flour is gluten-free and a great cooking option.

Rice milk - 0

Rice milk, made from milled rice and water, is typically gluten-free, but some strange ingredients tend to end up in store-bought plant milks so check the ingredients.

Rice noodles - 0

An excellent gluten-free option that often surprises people. Rice noodles, made from rice flour and water, are typically gluten-free. Always check labels to ensure they're not processed in a facility that handles gluten, or a product that contains gluten.

Rice paper - 0

Rice paper, made from rice flour, salt, and water, is typically gluten-free. An excellent alternative to wheat wraps.

Rice vinegar - 0

Rice vinegar, made from fermented rice, is typically gluten-free. Always check labels to ensure no gluten-containing additives are present.

Rosemary - 0

Runner beans - 0

Rutabaga, swede - 0

Rutabagas, also known as swedes, are gluten-free.

Rye - 2

Rye contains gluten. Should be avoided on a gluten-free diet.

Safflower oil - 0

Safflower oil is gluten-free.

Saffron - 0

Saffron is gluten-free.

Sage - 0

Salmon - 0

Sardines - 0

Sardines are gluten-free. However, if they are canned or prepared with sauces or marinades, these could contain gluten. It is a possibility, so always check labels.

Sauerkraut - 1

Sauerkraut is typically gluten-free as it's made from fermented cabbage. Always check labels to ensure there are no gluten-containing additives or extra ingredients.

Scallop - 0

Yes, gluten-free.

Sea bass - 0

Fine - gluten-free.

Sea bream - 0

Always gluten-free, watch out for sauces.

Seafood (fresh, unprocessed) - 0

Fresh, unprocessed seafood is gluten-free. Be cautious with processed or packaged seafood, as it could contain gluten-containing additives. Lots of fish sauces tend to be beautifully thick and creamy... and gluten-containing. So watch out for those.

Seaweed - 0

Seaweed is gluten-free.

Sesame oil - 0

Sesame oil is gluten-free, on its own.

Sesame seeds - 0

Sesame seeds are gluten-free.

Shallots - 0

Shallots are gluten-free.

Sheep - 0

Sheep meat, also known as lamb or mutton, is gluten-free, but look out for condiments, sauces and cooking methods.

Shiitake mushrooms - 0

Shiitake mushrooms are gluten-free.

Shrimp - 0

Shrimp is gluten-free, but look out for condiments, sauces and preparation methods.

Skimmed milk - 0

Skimmed milk is gluten-free.

Sloe berries - 0

Smoked fish (plain, no additives) - 0

Plain smoked fish with no additives is gluten-free - but ask if anything extra has been added in the smoking process.

Smoked meat (plain, no additives) - 0

A lot of smoked meat products do contain gluten. But plain smoked meat with no additives is gluten-free. Be cautious with flavored or pre-packaged smoked meats, which may contain gluten-containing additives.

Soba noodles - 2

Soba noodles are traditionally made from buckwheat, which is gluten-free, but our sources note they often also contain wheat flour. Therefore, they're not safe for those on a diet avoiding gluten, unless specifically labeled as gluten-free.

Sorbet - 1

Sorbet is typically gluten-free as it's usually made from fruit and sugar. However, some brands may use additives or thickeners that contain gluten, which is annoying, as you really would think it's just sugary frozen fruit liquid. Frustrating side note: Sometimes you'll ask for a gluten-free dessert in a restaurant, and they'll point blank tell you that all desserts have gluten in them. What odds they haven't bothered to check the sorbet ingredients!? Ask politely if they can look again.

Sorghum - 0

Sorghum is a grain that is gluten-free according to my sources. Many in our world love it as it is nutritionally dense and in fact gives more protein, iron, and numerous other vitamins and minerals than quinoa.

Sorghum flour - 0

See above. I like this - it's a good option. Sorghum flour, which is milled from sorghum grain, is gluten-free.

Soy sauce - 2

Ugh. Traditional soy sauce is made using wheat and is therefore not gluten-free. It also sneaks into various dishes and is a prime culprit. However, there are gluten-free versions available, often labeled as tamari sauce or gluten-free soy sauce.

Spaghetti squash - 0

Despite the name, spaghetti squash is a type of winter squash and is gluten-free safe.

Spinach - 0

Split peas - 0

Squash (all varieties) - 0

Star anise - 0

Star anise is gluten-free according to our expert sources.

Stevia - 0

Natural sweetener that should be gluten-free according to my sources. Good option for gluten-free baking.

Strawberries - 0

Yep, fine.

Sugar (white, brown, confectioner's) - 0

Pure sugar, whether white, brown, or confectioner's, is gluten-free. As always, check the label depending on how strict you are, as some brands may process their sugar in facilities that contain gluten.

Sunflower oil - 1

Sunflower oil should be gluten-free, but - very important - do not rely on sunflower oil in restaurants that has previously cooked other gluten-containing items. Ideally, a restaurant will have a separate fryer for gluten-free diners. Often you'll find there is a separate fryer for fries only.

Sunflower seeds - 0

Sunflower seeds are gluten-free.

Sweet potatoes - 0

Sweet potatoes are good, and an excellent kids gluten-free option for tea.

Swiss chard - 0

Swiss chard is a leafy green vegetable that is gluten-free.

Tangerines - 0

Tangerines are fine, gluten-free.

Tapioca - 0

Tapioca, from the root of the cassava plant, is gluten-free. Tapioca flour, also known as tapioca starch, is also gluten-free. It is another excellent baking option for gluten-free cooking, and particularly popular in various parts of the world including Brazil.

Tarragon - 0

Tarragon is a herb that is gluten-free.

Tea - 0

Pure, unflavored tea is gluten-free. However, flavored teas or teas with additives may contain gluten, so always check the label. Store bought tea drinks may also be fine, but check the label carefully.

Thyme - 0

Thyme is a herb that is gluten-free.

Tofu - 0

Plain, unflavored tofu is usually gluten-free. It's just made from soybeans. However, tofu can sometimes appear in strange forms. It can be flavored or processed tofu, and may contain gluten, so always check the label.

Tomatillos - 0

Tomatillos, a fave in Mexican cuisine, are gluten-free.

Tomatoes - 0

Tomatoes are fine, and gluten-free. Store-bought tomato sauces may not be. Gazpacho (a popular soup option) may sometimes contain gluten too.

Trout - 0

Tuna (fresh) - 0

Watch out for canned or packaged tuna contains gluten in the form of sauces, broth or other additives, so always check the label.

Turkey (fresh, unprocessed) - 0

Fresh natural turkey is fine. However, processed turkey products like sausages, patties, or deli meats may contain gluten, so always check the label or ask your butcher. In fact, most sausages do contain some form of gluten.

Turmeric - 0

Turmeric is no problem and gluten-free. Watch for additives.

Turnips - 0

Go turnip crazy. They're fine, as long as not combined with anything else.

Vanilla extract - 1

Pure vanilla extract is typically gluten-free. However, some lower quality or imitation vanilla extracts come in grain alcohol, so you do need to check the label.

Venison - 0

Venison, which is deer meat, is gluten-free.

Vinegar (distilled white, balsamic, wine, apple cider, but not malt) - 0

Distilled white vinegar, balsamic vinegar, wine vinegar, and apple cider vinegar are all gluten-free.

Important note, malt vinegar is not gluten-free as it's made from barley, a gluten-containing grain. That gets a big fat 2 on our scale.

Walnuts - 0

Watercress - 0

Watercress is absolutely fine.

Wheat - 2

Uh, that's why we're here, right? Wheat is a grain that contains gluten and should be avoided on a GF diet.

Wheatgrass - 2

Interestingly, the actual grass of wheatgrass does not contain any gluten. BUT (deep breath) it can be easily cross-contaminated with the wheat grain, which does contain gluten. So - the recommendation is to avoid wheatgrass unless it's specifically labeled as gluten-free. Ask at your juice bar for a guarantee that the wheatgrass they use is gluten-free.

Whitefish - 0

Wild rice - 0

Despite its name, wild rice is not actually rice but a type of grass. It is gluten-free.

Wine - 0

Fine. But watch out for store-bought wine mixers, coolers, and flavored wines which may contain barley malt.

Xanthan gum - 1

I urge caution. This is ordinarily gluten-free and often used in gluten-free baking. However, it can sometimes be derived from wheat, barley, or rye. Confusing. Try chia seed, egg, or tapioca starch as substitutes.

Yams - 0

A delicious, lesser-known carb substitute on the GF diet.

Yogurt (plain, unflavored) - 0

Typically gluten-free.

Zucchini - 0

We've spoken quite a bit about baking in this book. Some gluten-free bakers like to make Zucchini bread as an alternative to wheat based breads. Zucchini contains a lot of water so it makes your baking extra moist, which takes some practice but is delicious.

Made in United States
Orlando, FL
06 October 2024

52399933R00057